Livin' LaVida Grande:

Why You Can't Lose Weight

Raynette Ilg, N.D.

ISBN: 1496139224

ISBN-13:978-1496139221

DEDICATION

I would like to dedicate this book to
my wonderful husband Paul.

Paul is the man who went to learn how to cook, never
complained about cleaning, made the beds, did dishes and st
held down a rigorous job all because of his love for me while
went to school. It's his support and love that has allowed me
grow in my profession, laugh when it's good,
and laugh when it's tough.

I wish everyone had a spouse like him!

CONTENTS

INTRODUCTION

As you start to read this you will notice a few things. First of all I prefer to write the way I speak, so if you are looking for a book with sophisticated lingo, this isn't for you!

Secondly, I chose not to do a lot of annotating. I find it irritating at the very least when I'm reading a book and trying to get information. It makes me feel as if I have to have a degree in nuclear fission to get through the next paragraph!

Next, this book is not intended to treat anyone directly. This book is designed to give you ideas. Ideas about questions you have had so you can walk into your doctor's office, or better yet your Naturopath's office, and say "Hey, I did some reading and I know me best, this is what I believe is going on and why." I would even guess that if you are seeing a Naturopath they will be completely elated that you were doing some reading on your own because, guess what? A Naturopath understands that you know you best! What could be wrong with giving you the power? After all, you live with yourself 24/7. You know exactly what makes you tick!

Most people just need some good ol' fashioned guidance on how to make their health dreams come true. That's the goal of this book, and it's also the premise of Naturopathic care. As a matter of fact Naturopaths have a goal. It is to teach you how to take such great care of yourself that we might not be needed by you anymore!

Why did I write this? It just seems that there is always the latest and greatest fad to lose your tummy, reset your clock, be slim before summer, eat this way for only three weeks and you will be set for life, or buy our food that looks like the stuff you can't have!

I also love the infomercials showing a bunch of people who are just so happy since they have started the "Such and such program". Hmm, did you ever wonder what they look like five or ten years later? I do all of the time.

It just seemed to me that there were some

really basic things being overlooked. I mean, after all, the dieting industry is a multi-billion dollar industry, and for what? I would never shoot a mouse with an elephant gun if you know what I mean. Our society is filled to the gills with all kinds of microwave concepts. Which sounds better to you, a quick fix with a bad track record or a program of systemic change designed for you as an individual that is dedicated to optimizing your health?

Yes, weight loss is hard work.

Yes, you will need to learn some new skills and forget some old brain washing, but it will be worth more than you could ever imagine!

Sometimes correcting a nutrient deficiency or a change in eating habits can make all of the difference in the world. It can and has made many people the star of their own lives, that's what I want for you (quick, picture your name in lights!) If getting the basics balanced and changing the way you eat doesn't work, then, sure let's get into some of the bigger stuff...so you can be smaller.

CHAPTER 1

NATUROPATH

Mom, what's a Naturopath? Well, to answer that, let me explain how a Naturopath looks at things. So, what does it mean to take care of yourself naturally and use a natural health care practitioner to help? Does the image of a man wearing a multi-colored, tie-dyed shirt, long beard and sandals come to mind? If so, you're not alone. I think one of the stigmas that go along with natural care is the previously mentioned picture as well as the fear of being given some strange concoction that has floating leaves and twigs in it and tastes even worse.

Well, I'm here to tell you that those images aren't true at Olive Branch Wellness Center. Taking care of your health naturally, with the guidance of a natural health care professional, is a lot easier than you think and it can make a very large impact on how well you get through the winter, allergy season, mold season, or any season of your life, for that matter.

Principles

The principles that are followed for natural health care by a natural healthcare practitioner may seem quite simplistic, but when you really think about them, it changes your outlook on a lot of things. They are: First Do No Harm, Healing Power of Nature, Identify and Treat the Cause, Treat the Whole Person, Doctor as Teacher, and Prevention.

The first principle is: First Do No Harm. Now you're thinking, "That's right, do no harm, but everything is natural, so what's the big deal?" Well the big deal is this: too much of a good thing is exactly that, too much. For example, just because vitamin C is good for you doesn't mean you should be taking large quantities of it. High doses any vitamin can interfere with absorption of other vitamins, prescription medications, and processes which would then create a deficiency in something else and a new symptom for you to need to take an additional vitamin or herb.

Then the cycle begins. This is why it is good to get professional advice before you dive in; you may be healthier than you think to start with and not need what you think you need.

The second principle is: <u>The Healing Power of Nature</u>. Sounds kind of full of bologna, or should I say a big pile of tofu! Actually, your body is probably one of the finest machines you will ever own. The body, when given the proper nutrients, can overcome many obstacles and in fact it does on an hourly and daily basis. This basis to keep you going strong depends on what you need and what you already have nutrient wise. There are so many times in the course of a day that your body makes decisions without really consulting you. I guess you could say that in a strange way it doesn't need your approval to do what it has to do. You were born to follow a certain code and with proper nutrients your body will follow that code to maintain health when given the best opportunity and nutrients for health. You could say you have your own auto pilot!

The third principle is: <u>Identify and Treat the Cause</u>, also known as <u>Tonify the Weakened Systems</u>. We all have some area of the body that seems to take things the worst. How many times have you heard a friend say, "Every time I get sick it goes right to my chest!" or, "I can always tell when I'm going to get sick, I get (fill in the blank) first." Those are prime examples of weakened systems that might need support because they may be the gateway to you getting sick or just the system that needs tonifying.

This brings us to our next fine principle of taking care of your health, which is <u>Treating the Whole Person</u>. Sometimes we believe that treating the whole person is a no brainer, right? Wrong! Well then we think, "When I put a pill in, it treats everything, right?" Wrong! Each system of your body has particular food nutrient needs and vitamin and mineral needs. The irony is that if we are missing a particular vitamin in one area it changes things in other areas.

For instance, the mineral magnesium is responsible for over 300 chemical actions in the body. When we don't have enough magnesium, some strange things can happen such as sensitivity to sound and becoming irritable for no apparent reason. However, if the body has too much magnesium in the system, we can create diarrhea. (Please understand this is not meant to treat any condition, these are just examples of possibilities, nor is this a healthy way to diet!) So by taking a simple mineral, we have upset a delicate balance. So you can see how important it is to maintain nutrients because they truly do "treat the whole person".

Does any of this mean you should run out

and get a bottle of magnesium? No, it doesn't. Anyone who wants to start taking a supplement should be guided by a healthcare professional before they start to change the body chemistry and accidentally mistreat the whole body and interfere with their current prescriptions or health issues.

A Naturopathic healthcare practitioner is someone who, as one of our last points, Considers Him or Herself a Teacher. The best part of obtaining an appointment with a natural health care professional is that they will be teaching you how to best take care of your unique body for the cold and flu season and the conditions you have. Did you know that the more he or she teaches you about the care of your body, the less you will actually need him or her? That's an astonishing concept when you think about it, isn't it? Someone who is actually trying to put themselves out of business by taking care of you! All by teaching you to pay attention to the signs and signals your body gives you and how to respond to them will make your life better for the long run, and what could be better than that? I'll tell you what is better than that, our last principle, Prevention.

Prevention is where we all want to live, but let's face it; this prevention thing could take all of our time energy and a lot of money! Guess what: some of the best things for prevention are free! First of all, it's hard to attack a system that has been well rested. How about actually listening to your body and going to bed at a reasonable hour every night? Most of us want to accomplish so much that at the first sign of tiredness we push through it and get a second wind.

That second wind is dangerous. We end up staying up long after our body told us it just can't any more. We need sleep to allow all of our organs to rest and renew at the cellular level so they can fight the good fight and finish the race well every day. Prevention is one of the most important areas where your body will reward you with quality of life.

If you take care of the body, it will allow you to accomplish more than you could imagine. Through guided nutrition and supplementation everyone can have a better quality of life.

However you choose to take care of your health is up to you, but the most important thing is that you start now for a better year and a better quality of life.

NOTES

NOTES

CHAPTER 2

MINERAL DEFICIENCIES

Wouldn't it be great if all you had to do was just take one pill and it would even out everything in your body? Wait, didn't you think that's what your multi-vitamin would do? I know it's the dream we all have but heaven knows that's not a true reality for many Americans.

The truth is that deficiencies in different minerals can actually cause you to gain weight or at the very least impede your ability to lose weight efficiently. You see every time you go on one of the "latest and greatest" diets without having blood work done first to make sure your body is running in the optimal ranges, as opposed to functional ranges, you run the risk of depleting a mineral that is already just struggling to hang on in the body. So let's look at some of the basic minerals and discuss exactly what they do. Remember, your levels need to be checked first before you decide to start taking anything!

Magnesium

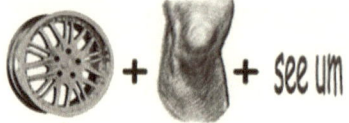 + see um

The first mineral I would like to discuss is magnesium. Over 50% of the magnesium in our body is found in our bones which makes magnesium is a real work horse in the body. Did you know it's the fourth most abundant mineral in the body? Without it many of the cycles of the body would cease to run. Magnesium is responsible for basically over 300 reactions in the body.

Those reactions include: anxiety and its friend nervousness, hormone balancing, muscle and nerve function, heart rhythm steadiness, a healthy immune system, regulation of blood sugar levels, protein synthesis, promotion of normal blood pressure, sleep quality, metabolism of both vitamins C and D, regulation of sodium and potassium, reduction of menstrual cramps, proper bowel function, and one of the big ones, stress and of course the list goes on!

Magnesium is primarily absorbed in the small intestine in two places and also, to a lesser degree, in the large intestine.

Magnesium also plays a large role in the production of hydrochloric acid in the stomach, which we all need in order to break food down for proper digestion and food utilization. Actually, magnesium also makes more energy by making more mitochondria, the powerhouse of each cell. Just think of the workouts you could be having if your magnesium is optimal.

As you can see, if the magnesium is off so is the rest of you! But more importantly some of the things you consume each day may actually deplete the body of this important mineral. Things like increased amounts of calcium and vitamin D3, and overindulgence in alcohol, caffeine, chocolate and sugar all increase the body's requirements for magnesium.

Some medications may also deplete the body of its precious magnesium as well. Medications such as diuretics and antibiotics deplete the magnesium from our system just to give a few. Also as we take a look at people who have some malabsorption issues such as Crohn's Disease, gluten sensitivity, and others who have chronic diarrhea syndromes like Irritable Bowel Syndrome, Irritable Bowel Disease, and still other people who have the wrong kind of harmful bacteria living in their intestines creating diarrhea.

Some people with chronically low amounts of potassium and calcium may also be suffering from low magnesium levels as well as the elderly, so you can see why a blood test is important to gaining insight for the magnesium level in your body.

The form of magnesium you take is important also. The most useable forms of magnesium in pill form or powder are aspartate, glycinate, or malate. Magnesium oxide is usually inexpensive but difficult for a lot of people to absorb so it might not get where it should go.

Then there is the use of Epsom salts in the bath water which is a great way to absorb magnesium into the system via your largest organ, the skin.

One of the other ways to get magnesium to enter the system quickly is via a Cell Salt called Mag phos. These are small little pills that can either go under the tongue or into a glass of water for quick absorption into the system, but remember only if you are tested and prove deficient in magnesium!

NOTES

NOTES

Calcium

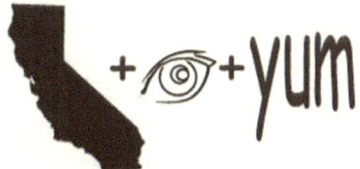 + 👁 + yum

Calcium is one of those things that we have been inundated with over the past few years.

Drink your milk, eat your veggies, take a calcium supplement, and get your calcium through this delightful chewy goodness and on and on. But what's the real deal with calcium and when is enough enough? Who do you believe? Don't I get enough in my multi-vitamin? My head is already spinning from too much calcium advertisement!

Your bones need most of your calcium; actually, 99% of it is stored in your bones. It's the other 1% which is the free calcium that we are concerned with because if there isn't enough of it someone is in trouble and that someone is you!

Calcium can actually regulate how fat is stored in the body. Personally I wouldn't like to have any fat storage, or at the very least have a say so in where it actually gets stored. I think I would like just a little here and a little there thank you. I like to jokingly think that if I need the fat I should be able to go on down to a big box store and get a bushel of it. But, alas, this is not the way it goes.

Calcium is known for its aid in the osteo's, such as osteopenia and osteoporosis, you know, the things you really don't want to have, or so they tell us on TV. Calcium is also extremely important in the function of numerous enzymes in the body. Especially the enzymes that break down nutrients into usable pieces for the body that would help with weight loss. Besides being a great bone builder, calcium also helps with the health of the heart, nerves, clotting of the blood, suppressing hunger, reducing blood pressure, PMS, teeth health, central nervous system health (i.e. the brain), and muscles and the impulses between them.

One of the very unique things about the body and calcium is that the body will steal calcium from the bones in order to run its other processes efficiently if there isn't enough free calcium. That in turn leaves your weight loss and bones in a large predicament.

Calcium also needs other minerals and vitamins in order to be absorbed such as vitamin D, zinc and magnesium as well as vitamin K. Some of the vitamins and minerals that compete for the same receptor sites as calcium are: iron, manganese and copper so they shouldn't be taken when calcium is taken otherwise no one is happy. One of the things we need to consider is that estrogen plays an important role in helping to increase calcium absorption so sometimes that is a big factor, and yes, that can be a problem if you are a male, too!

Some foods actually aid in the depletion of calcium from the body such as salt and excessive amounts of protein. Caffeine is also a culprit of calcium depletion (I know, there goes your coffee and chocolate again!) Then there are the foods that can diminish the amount of calcium you absorb like: beans, soybeans, nuts, spinach, sweet potatoes, certain teas and wheat bran.

As we talked about in the section on magnesium, certain drugs can deplete calcium as well. Medications like: antacids, corticosteroids, antibiotics, diuretics, osteoporosis medications, asthma medications, and ulcer medications.

At the risk of sounding redundant if you have malabsorption issues then chances are you need to get your calcium checked as well because it's probably not going to be where you think it is!

So now we come to which form of calcium is best? I always say the food form is best, dark green leafy vegetables or maybe some bone in salmon but what if you don't like those? Calcium citrate is one of the easiest for the body to absorb because it does not require extra stomach acid to dissolve and it is known for being less irritating to the intestinal wall than other forms of calcium. Face it you won't take it if you feel nauseous after taking it the first time.

Calcium carbonate has a higher percentage of elemental calcium in it and is the most common calcium found on the market today, however the molecule is extremely large and required additional stomach acid in order to be broken down in to usable pieces. There are many ways to get your calcium. Liquids, pills, powders, and cell salts, but remember to be tested before you run out and start downing calcium.

Be aware that antacids are not a good way to get your daily calcium so no matter how delicious some of them taste, step away from the bottle!

NOTES

NOTES

Zinc

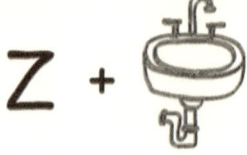

Really, zinc? Yes, zinc!

Most people only think of zinc for a cold, but not true. Zinc is great, only if you need it. What in the world does it do? You see we know about calcium and we kind of know about magnesium, but what in the world do we know about zinc?

The answer is, you probably are thinking long and hard right about it now, so let me put you out of your misery.

Zinc is necessary for all kinds of good old immune functions so basically anything that ends in "itis". Good for: wound healing, sensory perception (where you are in time), fat burning hormones of the thyroid, and leptin (the hormone that both increases energy and tells the brain your stomach is full), increases your metabolic rate, necessary for proper taste and smell, healthy sperm, testosterone production, and renewal of hair, skin, nails, and vision.

You can find good sources of zinc in meat, nuts and seafood. Zinc, however, is required for enzymatic reactions, so basically someone needs someone else so they can get their job started!

A lot of the reactions for your thyroid hormone, which we all secretly hope is the reason we have gained weight, require zinc to start the action. Since the thyroid plays a pretty big role in regulating your metabolism we want to make sure it's doing everything it can to help us burn those calories.

One of the other benefits of zinc is that it can greatly enhance something called leptin. Leptin is one of those hormones that helps to enhance the use of your energy and who wouldn't want more of that! Leptin also has a unique signaling system and tells you brain that you're full, so stop eating. At this point it's simple math; eat less = smaller you.

Some of the more common drugs that deplete zinc in your body are: Anti-inflammatories (inhalants, systemic and topical corticosteroids), ACE Inhibitors, aluminum, NSAIDS, some birth control medications, diuretics and ulcer medications.

Well, now that you are either depressed or grabbing your coat and wallet to fly to the store and get some zinc, take a breath and think. Do you know for sure if you need zinc? If the answer is I didn't have a blood test to check, then get back in your chair and don't take zinc until you have been told to!

Remember, too much of a good thing is still too much.

Well let's say you actually find out you do need zinc, what kind should it be? Like many other supplements there are certain forms that are a little bit more beneficial than others.

Take for instance there is the zinc picolinate which you can find on most shelves at the store. This form of zinc is actually chelated which means that it has been through the chelation process and the molecules have been given an electrical charge that will allow them to positively attract the zinc mineral which in turn creates a temporary increase in the concentration of the mineral inside the molecule. This process lets the mineral attach to something else like an amino acid (I like to think of it like potato chips adhere to my hips!) This chelation, in theory, gives the body a better chance to absorb the mineral. The jury is still out on this!

Zinc orotate is probably the best. This form is also a chelated form of zinc but this time chelated to orotic acid. This orotic acid is a form that the body really likes and so it is absorbed easier and put into the cells quicker.

The last form is a zinc gluconate. It's a pretty popular form of zinc but remember transforming zinc into a gluconate is done through an industrial manufacturing process that uses a fermentation of glucose which gives the product a longer shelf life.

My money would be on the zinc orotate if I needed it, but remember to be tested first! There's nothing like taking something and then creating a problem because you really didn't need it to start with!

NOTES

NOTES

CHAPTER 3

VITAMIN DEFICIENCIES

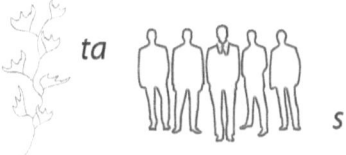 ta s

Vitamins Overview

So now we come to a different part of the "Grande" story where I want to talk about vitamins. One of the questions I hear all of the time is, "Should I take a multi-vitamin?" Well yes, I believe you should! I believe it is necessary because you never really know on any given day how much of a vitamin your body may be plowing through for its functions. I mean, after all, there isn't really a meter on your forehead saying, "Danger, Danger, low on Vitamin C today!"

A good quality multi-vitamin can do wonders for keeping things running at a base line. Then there is the problem of "What if I'm low on a vitamin that's already in my multi, then what?"

Well, then, I believe you should talk to a natural healthcare provider to see what you should take and exactly how much and for how long!

The reasons for your body chewing through that vitamin or mineral quicker than you can put it in might be something someone who knows more than you should be consulted with for good measure. A lot of times you just might need a little extra to get you up to par! I liken it to a bucket that has a hole in it and you are trying to fill it with a thimble. You have two choices in this situation; either use a bigger thimble or work faster! It works much the same way with vitamins.

All of that said, vitamins are different from minerals. I know you never really gave that much thought and you now think, hey, my minerals are in my vitamins, but let's really talk about the difference.

Vitamins are organic which means that they can be broken down by things such as heat, acids, or air. Minerals on the other hand are considered inorganic. Minerals will hold onto their structure no matter what!

So exactly where do we find minerals? Well minerals can be found in many places like soil and water. The minerals then find their way to you via plants, fish, animals and the liquids you drink. The body then absorbs them along the digestive pathway.

Vitamins have a little bit of a tougher time getting into the body. This difficulty happens because of the way we treat food. When we cook food, a lot of the nutrients get lost in either the water or the over cooking of the food, or the actual way we cook the food, you know, like the microwave.

Now make sure you understand I'm not telling you to run out and eat everything raw. Yuck! I'm just making the statement that some things need to be compensated for or if they can be changed easily then

let's change them for the better.

So here are some of the "Grande" vitamins that may be missing in your body and contributing to "Livin' La Vida Grande."

NOTES

NOTES

Vitamin C

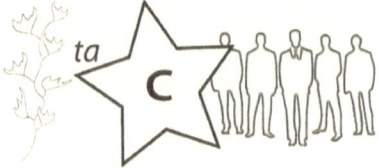

Vitamin C is one of the cooler vitamins in my book! It has a great relationship with all of the glands. Vitamin C is another big hitter and is responsible for at least three hundred metabolic functions in the body. How cool is that!

Vitamin C is used by the body for tissue growth and tissue repair, adrenal function (those stressed out adrenal glands just love them some Vitamin C), healthy gums, strengthening the immune system, asthma, increases the absorption of iron, reducing LDL's (that's the bad cholesterol), increasing HDL's (the good cholesterol), necessary for the formation of collagen, for good elasticity in both the skin so it all goes back when you lose the weight and for the little smooth muscles inside of your arteries to promote a healthy blood pressure, protects against abnormal blood clotting and bruising, not to mention promoting the healing of wounds and burns, joint pains, poor digestion and certain kinds of tooth loss. Vitamin C attacks free radicals in the body's biologic fluids. Since the body can't make Vitamin C, it counts on us to get the Vitamin C we need through either foods or supplements.

So which drugs deplete Vitamin C? Well here you go; birth control pills, analgesics, antidepressants, anticoagulants, diabetic medications, and certain steroids. Some of the other things that we consume just for fun suck the Vitamin C out of our systems as well. Things like alcoholic beverages and smoking! Who would have thought smoking and alcohol take a toll in a new way! But then again, somewhere in the back of your mind you kind of already knew that right, right?

So what is the best form of Vitamin C to take? Yikes, there are so many of them! Well, how about this? Why don't I give you the information and see what you do with it? By the way, it's not orange juice, so boo hoo, you have no reason to drink the sugary stuff!

So here's the big deal. There are pretty much two types of Vitamin C.

The first one is calcium ascorbate and the second one is ascorbic acid. Here's the difference between the two. First of all, the different types of Vitamin C matter because of the ph of your blood. Some people are just a little more acidic in their blood ph (not the saliva ph or the urine ph). Blood ph runs close to 7.46 and that's the ph that most people will achieve optimal absorption for Vitamin C and other vitamins too!

So wait, how do you know which one to take? Well if you are on the more acidic side of things calcium ascorbate will be your new friend. If you are a little more basic (not in the head, in the ph!) you will do better with ascorbic acid.

Then there is the problem of what do you know about Ester-C©? Here's the deal on it. Ester - C© is mainly calcium ascorbate. There are some other smaller forms of molecules that are other things but this form of Vitamin C has no greater absorption than the basics so this may be the best time to stick with the basics for your best health.

Whether you chose the calcium ascorbate or the ascorbic acid form make sure you take it in divided doses. Dividing up the doses insures that your body will make use of it rather than look at it, say "I have enough" and dump the rest.

NOTES

NOTES

Vitamin D

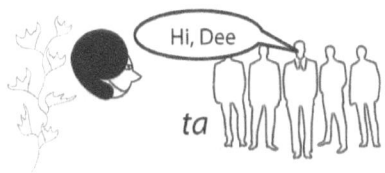

Wow, look at the tan on that guy! Well yes, look at him. The real skinny is, "What's his Vitamin D level?" Maybe now you're thinking "Well I don't really care what *his* Vitamin D level is and why should I?" Well, if it's someone you are related to you should care, but even more so, what's yours? Some of the misconceptions about a tan person or someone of Mediterranean descent is that they must already have enough Vitamin D! Guess what it might not be true! Shocked? Yeah, well, I was too the first time I saw the labs on a nice tan person.

Vitamin D is basically one of the newer kids on the block. Lately there has been a lot of research about Vitamin D and what your levels should be and exactly what it's used for in the body. First of all Vitamin D is a hormone, but we call it a vitamin. There are two ways to get Vitamin D in you.

Vitamin D is a fat soluble vitamin, so that means it needs to be absorbed with fat in order for the body to recognize it and use it. The first way we get Vitamin D is from sunlight. Vitamin D is transferred into the body through the skin with sunlight via cholesterol to an inactive form of Vitamin D. The inactive form then travels through the body first to the liver and then to the kidneys where it is turned into the active form of Vitamin D.

The second way to get Vitamin D is to get it through supplementation (you know, pills!)

Vitamin D is necessary in the body for many functions including; reducing the risk of colon polyps, prostate cancer, decreased coronary artery disease, decreased chance of developing Type 1 diabetes, weight reduction, bone density, multiple sclerosis, pregnancy health, muscle strength, immune function, asthma, rickets, increase the risk of fibroids, helps with irritable bowel syndrome, acne, depression, tooth decay, and high blood pressure.

Medications that deplete Vitamin D are the following; mineral oil taken internally, orlistate (the over the counter weight management drug that keeps you from absorbing fat!), laxatives antacids, anti-seizure medications, some cholesterol lowering drugs, and ulcer medications. If you are taking any of these you may need to have a Vitamin D level taken to ensure that you are holding enough Vitamin D in your body for proper function!

So what form should you take? Well there are two types.

The first one is a Vitamin D2 type which is called ergocalciferol which comes from food type sources.

The second type is Vitamin D3 (cholecalciferol) which synthesized or changed in the skin in response to exposure to the sun's ultraviolet rays. The sun type form is typically considered the best form to obtain whether it is in supplement form or from real honest to goodness sun rays.

Now hear this, I am not saying roast all day outside in the sunlight and damage your skin beyond recognition, what I am saying is that a combination of sunlight and supplementation is usually the best for your body.

NOTES

NOTES

Vitamin B *Complex*

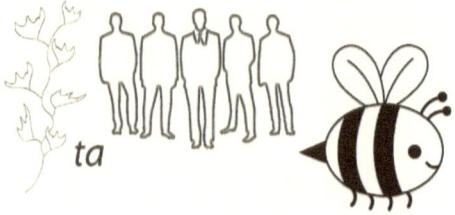

ta

So what I've noticed is that there is a lot of confusion out there about B complex vitamins. Some people think that just taking one B vitamin such as B12 is the same as taking a B complex. Wrong! There are B vitamins numbered up to B17! A typical B complex will contain B vitamins up to B12 and include things such as PABA, biotin, choline and inositol, weird words you see on the label and think, yeah, whatever, I must need it otherwise it wouldn't be in there!

B vitamins have a fun claim to fame. B vitamins when they pass through or should I say out of you make your urine that bright yellow that freaks everyone out! The reason they turn your urine bright yellow has to do with the riboflavin's (B2) chemical reaction in your body. It's okay, you aren't dying! B vitamins are water soluble and go directly into the blood. When the riboflavin gets to the kidneys they find the excess riboflavin and send it packing, hence the bright yellow urine. Well here is the other thing. If you are low in one B vitamin typically you are low in them all. Why? Because B vitamins are known for working in a team like fashion and breaking one down to make another until there is no more to break down.

Do you remember the statement I made earlier about taking a multi-vitamin because you don't know what you're going to need on a daily basis? Well the same thing applies if you need B complex vitamins. So exactly what do they do? Here's the list and I'll warn you its quite impressive! (long, too, but read it anyway!)

B vitamins do the following: maintain the health of nerves (kinda good if you've got someone on them!) skin, eyes, hair, liver and mouth: muscle tone; gastrointestinal tract; brain function (don't think I don't know what you're thinking here!); help enzymes react with other substances; energy; depression; anxiety; dementia; enhance circulation; assist in blood formation; carbohydrate metabolism; production of hydrochloric acid; muscle tone of the intestines, heart and stomach; protect from aging; effects from drinking and smoking; antibody production; cell growth; helps with the use of oxygen in the tissues of the skin, nails, and hair; eliminates dandruff; helps the absorption of iron; helps with the absorption of other B vitamins; metabolism of fats and proteins; normal secretion of bile; lower cholesterol; synthesis of sex hormones; reduction of canker sores; diarrhea; dizziness: fatigue; bad breath; headaches; insomnia; low appetite; (I know, that's not the reason you are reading this book!) low blood sugar; and decreases stress. Are you tired of the list yet? I am! Phew!

So now we come to the ever important, "What's the best form to take?" Hmm, let's see. First of all they come in different dosages. Most come either 50mg or 100mg.

You should only take the 100mg if you are under the supervision of a qualified health care professional. Self diagnosis equals bad diagnosis!

Secondly, there should be useable forms of the B vitamins in the complex.

Things like niacin, not niacinamide, methylcobalamin for B12 and not cyanocobalamin. Forms that have a co-enzymated process so the body can quickly and efficiently absorb the vitamins and help to get you thin more quickly, right?

Also pass by any brand that has artificial colorings or dyes. If you are trying to get healthy why would you want to gum it up with artificial stuff! It sounds as if the forms of B vitamins are easier to pick out, and they may be, just keep the previous guidelines in place and you will urinating yellow in no time at all!

NOTES

NOTES

CHAPTER 4

Other Stuff

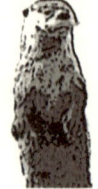 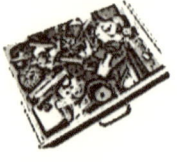

Argh! You mean there's other stuff! Yep. Some of the "Other Stuff" can be some of the hardest stuff to do. You know, things you kind of already know but don't really want to admit to or do!

Sweeteners

Let's talk about the first one, sugar reduction. Yes I know it's kind of like air, its everywhere! Once you get the taste of sugar your body naturally wants more. The more places we consume sugar the less sensitive to sweetness we actually become.

What that ends up meaning is that it takes more and more of a sweetener to actually convince the tongue and the brain that what you are eating is sweet. It's the over abundance of sugar and its other forms that starts changing your form! Most people will find that if they can be strict and eliminate sugar in all forms for three months they will look in the mirror and wonder who that skinny person is and where did they stuff the rest!

Now here comes the big problem, we think that we can just substitute fruit in the place of all of the sugar we want to eat.

Well, some low glycemic fruits, yes, but not that big ol' bowl full of fruit because, "it's healthy, right?" Here's the thing. Too much of a good thing is still too much. The amount of low glycemic fruit you should consume per day is 2 cups, max. In case you are wondering how much that really is, 1 apple is about 1 cup. Yeah, I know! All you people who are over eating fruit, raise your hands!

What about your favorite grande non fat (non fat does not necessarily equal healthy), triple mocha, frappe something or other. Are you aware that most of those drinks have an excess of 40 grams of sugar per drink! I know what you're thinking. Yes, they are delicious, but really, do you need that much sugar? Ah, no.

Next is my absolute, favorite, the "Sports Drink." Most of those are in the too much sugar and we aren't even going to talk about the additives and coloring agents! I don't know about you but I really can't find any fruit that naturally is that color blue!

Do we really need to talk about pop, I mean, really!

Don't sit there and think, "well, its diet!" Yes, I know, but it's just as bad for you if not worse. There are the artificial sweeteners that are added to them to make them diet. You don't need pop to live or breathe!

Basically, we don't need the donuts, bagels, hunks of gooey or crusty bread, pizza dough, pancakes or other things that have sugars in them either. (Boo!)

I just want to let you know that honey is not a good healthy alternative either. Honey has a really high glycemic index and load, which equals sugar! By the way, so does agave syrup.

What can you sweeten with? Well, stevia, and real stevia from the health food store, not the stuff you get in the grocery store aisle that begins with a T, is great to use. It doesn't mess with your liver the way that fructose does. You see fructose has to be handled differently in the body.

Glucose, regular sugar is handled by the cells in your body, every cell to be exact, and consequently is burned up almost immediately after you consume it. Glucose stores much less of its end product as fat, usually less than one calorie!

Fructose, on the other hand, is turned into free fatty acids and some bad cholesterol and triglycerides, or as we may be able to see, fat! You see, when you consume fructose, then the processing burden is on the liver, and that means extra work for it.

So now let's move on from sugar now that you are completely bummed out!

After sugar, let's talk about portion control.

Most of us like to feel a little full, I know I do. But really, how much is enough? Just because we finished the most fabulous meal of our life and now they are bringing out dessert, do you really need it? Think twice about that. Are you going to be running a marathon tomorrow and burn off those extra calories? Yeah, me neither.

Sometimes one of the best things to happen to a person is to fall down and break both arms so your hands can't get to your mouth!

(This is not a treatment suggestion!) Look at the food on your plate. I mean really look at it. Now look at your fist. Your stomach is about the size of your fist. How much of what is on the plate will equal your fist? Do you need a mound of that food or will a couple of bites give your hungry taste buds what they need? Rethink...... yes your fist!

Your stomach can expand if you really need it to, but my question is should you be forcing it to expand at every meal or only rarely? Just think of the money you will save on groceries if you only ate the amount of food that is the size of your fist!

I know if you have been eating lots of ooey gooey sugary good stuff that has increased your appetite, your stomach will be mad at you for trying to decrease your portions, but I have news for you, it will get over it!

What your body will do is look around inside itself and decide to start breaking down that extra butt you have been carrying around and what could be bad about that?

NOTES

NOTES

Social Eating

Hmm, so are you a social eater?

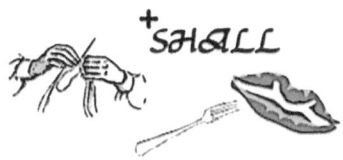

You know the time you are sitting there with some friends and there is a big plate of nachos sitting there and then all of a sudden they are gone and you think, "no, it can't be! Did I eat that whole thing?" Yes that person. Is that you? If it is, you might need to do some early damage control. How about you sit far away from the food or make it difficult to reach? I know those seem like simplistic measures but trust me you will feel pretty awkward about eating something if you have to knock people down to do it!

Do you think when you go out you should just cheat and let it all hang out? You know what I mean, "Oh, oops the chicken had double the sauce on it!" or, "hmm, there isn't anything I can really eat here so it's either go big or go home!"

Well, I don't believe it. Most of the restaurants can make food without the sauce or they have enough selections that you can get something without the messy bad stuff on it! I really guess it comes down to how committed you are. Are you committed or do you need to be committed?

I used to think when I ate at someone's home that no matter what they served I had to eat what they had the way they served it. You know over the years I've found that people aren't really concentrating on what's on my plate as much as they are interested in having good conversation and having fun.

You can always find a way to modify what they are serving, always! Take for instance spaghetti. I don't do well with noodles so I just ate sauce on my lettuce and I was perfectly happy! My hostess even tried it and she liked it too. I also find that many people are serving lighter meals and even lighter desserts. I mean really, how many pudding/jello/cookie/cake things can you really eat? Most people are asking for just a little piece and they are satisfied, you should too!

Now, under this category I'm going to put a very important issue and don't misunderstand what I'm saying about this subject, *Closet Eating*.

Do you think to yourself "That will be my treat when he or she is gone or in bed?" Why? Are you ashamed to eat it in front of other people? Do you think that they won't notice the bag of candy, chips or popcorn is gone and you're passed out on the couch?

Fess up! Sometimes the best thing you can do is tell someone that you don't want to eat that so they should take it out of the house and then guess what? Don't buy it again! No, you don't need to have it on hand for the kids, the guests or just in case. The truth of the matter is you know down deep you are going to eat it no matter what!

Be honest with yourself; it seems like a silly statement but you might even like yourself a little more when you are! This actually brings me to the next section of the book.

NOTES

NOTES

Hormones

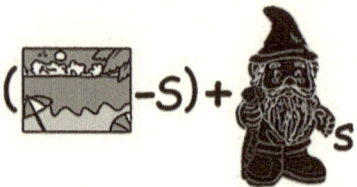

Do you think that sometimes no matter how hard you try your body can override everything and make you do something? (That is not an excuse!) Well, so do I! Now I bet you are really relieved, I was too! We know that men and women both have testosterone, progesterone and estrogen. It's just the amounts of each that differs. If you are a male reader, don't skip this section. You have the same problem so we will start with you first.

So what do you know about testosterone other than the obvious? Well here is the deal. Testosterone is used for many things in the male body. Do you know what they are? Here is the list: sharper mind, better mood, increased muscle mass and strength (which will equal better fat burning capabilities), a healthier heart, stronger libido, stronger bones and good clean energy, better fat distribution, red blood cell production, and sperm production, deeper voice, thicker hair shafts, and larger organs. And you just thought it was for one thing... growing a beard, right?!

With all of that said, it is important to make sure if you are a male that your testosterone is optimal! One positive result of corrected testosterone levels is the increased probability of living longer. However, if it isn't optimal then you could be experiencing the big ol' beer belly. This beer belly tends to appear in response to changing levels of testosterone.

When testosterone dips then the stomach starts to get bigger and the fat deep under the skin and around the organs starts to increase. The next thing after that is the heart can start to experience circulatory problems, like increased blood pressure and an increase in the triglyceride level. We've already talked about triglycerides!

This abdominal fat usually has a direct relationship with insulin resistance and something called metabolic syndrome. Both of those are not good, in case you were wondering. Just think: closer to diabetes.

Once those take hold it's pretty hard to get rid of them! Talk about work! I think it would be easier to keep in shape earlier than worry about the fallout later!

The problem is that many of the chemicals in food begin to disrupt the hormones and their signaling and then we begin to have problems. For you men, the estrogen receptors can get activated and stay that way.

What does that mean to you? One of the problems can be weight gain. This particular weight gain is due to incorrect feedback loop signaling, perhaps better thought of as turning something on that needs to stay off!

Another issue is higher than normal glucose (still not good!).

Still another side effect, prostate cancer, also not good!

Then there are the very picturesque Moobs! (Man boobs)

Something else can happen, too. I know, what, there's more? Yes, there is. The feel good hormones can take a turn for the worst. We will discuss that one in the next chapter.

Now, then, how about the women out there? Yeah sometimes I think that balancing hormones for a woman is like riding a schizophrenic horse towards a burning barn!

Men only have one hormone and basically either it's turned on or off. Women however have hormones that look like the dashboard of an airplane! On any given day at any given time things can look totally different than they did an hour ago. So, here goes.

Women's major hormone is estrogen, right? Some women become more sensitive to estrogen and have a higher amount than necessary of it in the system, also, not good.

This higher amount can make a woman more susceptible to cancers, skipped menstrual periods, decreased mental ability, endometriosis, infertility, heart disease, stroke, water retention, irregular bleeding, headaches, breast pain, weight gain, promote blood clot formation, enlarged breasts, changes in body temperature, and an increase of cholesterol.

Additionally, women may have a higher amount of estrogen caused by not having enough progesterone. Either way this should be checked out by a healthcare professional!

NOTES

NOTES

Neurotransmitters

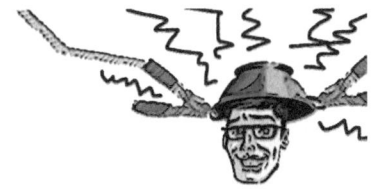

The thing is, whether you are male or female, the hormonal control mechanism is up higher than you think it is. It's in the brain. Sometimes it is a matter of getting the brain chemistry balanced out to help you keep your weight under control. You see serotonin has its main residence in the gut, where 90% of your body's is located. That's why eating certain foods can make you feel oh so good! Some of the rest of it is in the brain, or as it's better known, the central nervous system.

So let's talk about serotonin first. We all tend to think about it as the "feel good, I'm not depressed" hormone. There are so many other functions of serotonin. It helps with regulation of your mood, constriction of the blood vessels, appetite, a little bit of the sleep, memory, some responsibility for learning, regulation of insulin and growth factor, sexual behavior, body temperature and hormonal system. Of course we are going to be more concerned with the stuff hanging around the central nervous system and the gut here as it pertains to regulation of insulin and growth factor.

The next neurotransmitter on the list is dopamine. Released by the brain it is involved in pleasurable reward, memory, attention, movement, Parkinson's Disease, drug addiction, erections, and facial tics. I think we are going to use this one for its pleasurable reward function although I have to admit I was thinking that the memory of whether or not you just ate the bag of candy or chips was second in my thoughts!

Dopamine gives you that energy or kind of a boost to get you up and doing the things you should be doing and then helps you to keep doing them by giving you increased focus, better concentration. All that and how about a scoop of better memory?!

Really, serotonin and dopamine work together to help control your sense of appetite and those uncontrollable cravings for sweets and other carbs, especially those things like bagels and pasta and cookies, oh my!

The third neurotransmitter is norepinephrine. Well, it's a hormone and a neurotransmitter. Norepinephrine has a big role in the body. One of its more famous roles is that it affects the heart during times of stress. What it does is it increases the rate of contractions of the heart during times of the ol' "Fight or Flight" response to stressors, you know like when you are being chased by a bear!

It can play a big part in making your adrenal glands work over time and let's face it, most of us don't like working overtime and your adrenal glands are the same way. Then there is the problem of getting the surge of stress all the time which leads us to having too much cortisol in the system and that equals a big belly!

So how do those neurotransmitters get all mixed up and running in the wrong direction? Easy enough to comment on, but not necessarily easy enough to wrangle around with a firm answer.

First of all there can be some damage to them because of stress. Stress either by physical damage or from some toxic junk that can wreak havoc on the system.

Secondly, there just might be some nutrients missing. Remember when I was talking earlier about getting your vitamins and minerals straightened out? Well this is a good reason to get going on that.

Thirdly, maybe you just got a set of crummy genes and you will need to get some of the neurotransmitters straightened out. Any way you slice it neurotransmitters are a huge part of being able to lose weight.

Some of the foods that can enhance neurotransmitters are also some of the foods that can cause some weight gain if you are thinking you can really feed yourself back to optimal neurotransmitters, I would think again.

Especially since the quantities of those foods would set you up for Olympic eating should you decide to take that route to a neurotransmitter balance.

There are also medications that tend to reduce serotonin. Things like; diet pills, pain killers, and recreational drugs. Then there are the medications and other things that lower dopamine. Things like; toxic chemicals such as PCBs, certain amounts of carbohydrates, low levels of iron and zinc and B vitamins.

Then there's the estrogen deficiencies in women not to mention the abusive consumption of alcohol and narcotics. Now what about norepinepherine? Well that one can be lowered by; certain anti-depressants, blood pressure medications, and some of the main heart medications.

So by now you can see that this is not an area you should be navigating by yourself, but an area you should be seeking help from a professional about!

Neurotransmitters can really make a difference in your weight and overall sense of well being, however it's not for you to treat. Get help! This isn't "Neurotransmitters for Dummies." Get it? LOL!

NOTES

NOTES

CHAPTER 5

POINTING AT THE INNARDS!

Let's start pointing fingers! Yeah, that's it! I think we will start pointing fingers at the digestive system first, how does that strike you?

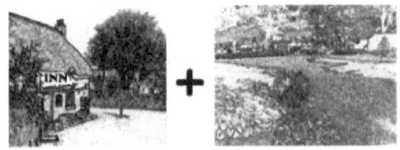

Digestive Issues

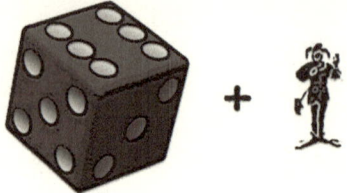

Digestion is both a complicated process and a non-complicated process. First of all, nothing is inside your body (even if you eat it) until it is digested and passes through the membranes of your intestines into the bloodstream!

So basically you are just one big long tube from mouth to anus. Please, no extra added comments here from me! It is the enzymes, good bacteria and to some smaller extent, vitamins and minerals that play a part in getting the food you eat past this membrane, into the system and ready for use in your body. But what if there is a problem? What if you have issues that don't allow you to get that food rockin', rollin' and a' churnin'? What would those things be? What would that feel or look like?

Here are some of the more common things that get in the way of you getting all you can from your food in the digestive tract. Here are some of the biggies; Gluten intolerance, food allergies, bad bacteria hanging around in the digestive tract that you picked up who knows where, lack of good bacteria and finally: yeast.

I'll start with gluten intolerance/celiac disease. For these people grains other than corn, rice, spelt, kamut, some oats, amaranth, buckwheat, millet, teff, and sorghum spell trouble. Bouts of diarrhea, vomiting, itching and even constipation can make them miserable. As a matter of fact, I think those things would make any of us miserable. The fact that they have aggravated their digestive tract then causes the malabsorption of vitamins and minerals, hence back to the beginning!

Gluten intolerance is a miserable disease and initially should be closely managed by a professional who is very familiar with it so you can get the right advice on foods and nutritional deficiencies. Please realize that I could go on for quite a while on gluten intolerance but this book is not totally about gluten intolerance so we are going to have to move on!

Here we are at food allergies. Food allergies are usually fun little buggers! When most of us think about allergies we think about runny noses, red eyes, or big honkin' welts on the body that are red. Well, some of that may be true but not the only way your body expresses an allergy. I think I will use myself as an example since I can't talk about you.

First of all I have four allergies: Chicken, corn, rice and eucalyptus. Who would ever think that a person can be allergic to chicken! Well I am. When I eat chicken I get short of breath, my hands, feet and knees hold fluid for days and I could scratch through my skin and down to the bone and then right on down through the bone to China! So my question to you is did you notice that my hands, feet and knees hold fluid?

Yep, fluid in the wrong spots equals weight gain. Maybe you should really think about what you believe is healthy and see what it does to you. This does not mean avoid vegetables, fruits and other healthy things in case you're wondering. There is no cheese doodle diet!

Corn on the other hand makes me very, very grumpy. No not grumpy, just down right mean. That means that my system isn't clearing it so it's hanging around. Corn is one of the biggest reasons for weight gain. Not only is it a huge carbohydrate but the body just can't seem to digest it and get rid of it. You know what I'm talking about because after you eat an ear of corn, what do you see in the toilet the next day? Whole pieces of corn! It just doesn't break down.

Then there is rice. I know you're thinking what does she mean she's allergic to rice? Rice makes me sleep for hours. ¼ cup of rice and I'm out for the count! So it goes to figure that eating rice and sleeping afterwards does nothing for burning off the carbohydrates or calories in rice which in the long run equals a bigger dent in the couch where I fall asleep!

How do you take care of this? Well there's expensive testing that can be done, there are elimination diets, food journals and scratch tests. Any way you slice it there are ways to figure it out! Just get it figured out. The funny thing is a lot of times, not always, but a lot of times its going to be something you are constantly eating! Don't be a baby, just get it figured out.

Let's just take some time now and talk about bad bacteria. So there are thousands of kinds of bacteria in your intestines that work together on every scrap of food you put in, to break it down and get it past the membrane of your intestines and into your bloodstream so you can use it. But what if you've gotten some bad bacteria somewhere?

Where could that come from, pray tell? Anywhere really, a salad bar with things that were starting to turn or lettuce that hasn't been properly washed, people not washing their hands after using the bathroom (ewww!), bacteria on door knobs or money, basically anywhere. What happens is this bad bacteria sets up camp in the intestines and starts to push out the good bacteria and then makes you miserable! By miserable I mean diarrhea, stomach pains, constipation, overly hungry, overly sleepy, or not able to absorb nutrients.

What's a person to do about this? Get a stool test, but get one that asks questions the right way. Sometimes you will go to the doctor's office and they will get a stool sample from you and ask the lab if the top three or four bacterias are there. That's nice, but not the right question. You see the right question is not "Is this, this, or this there?" The right question is, "Show me what is there." Sometimes people have the darnedest things hanging around in there and those are the things we need to find. Also we do a culture and sensitivity test to show what kills what's there. I mean what good does it do to know what is there if you don't know what will kill it?

I'm only gonna say this once. If you don't have enough good bacteria, then you have too much bad bacteria. Think about it. Take a minute before we move on.

Yeast. We need yeast in our systems in order for them to function. It is however the overabundance of yeast that is the problem. Yeast can make you itchy, irritable, fat, pimply, and throw just about everything you eat out of whack in terms of digestion.

Yeast loves sugar and the over abundance of breads, pastas, cookies, crackers, rice, potatoes, candy, pop, alcoholic beverages, all the sweet drinks you get at the coffee shops and the "good for you smoothies" you love to get because you think you're gonna get healthy. Here's the deal. Yeast is a beast! It lives inside you driving you to run for the candy dish on your co-worker's desk. It drives you to donuts, pie, cake, loads of fruit, anything you can get your sweet little mitts on, even cough drops!

If you think you might have a yeast problem you will truly need a stool test because yeast cultures will be part of what is analyzed. Once the yeast is properly killed off you will be surprised at how your weight changes for the better.

Now, don't misunderstand what I'm saying here. I am not saying run to the health food store and buy something tomorrow for yeast. What I am saying is, get tested for yeast. You can do damage if you start taking even natural things if you don't need them. Repeat after me, "I will not try this on my own no matter what I see on TV or what the health food store employee tells me".

So let's sum this section up in four words.

Get your digestion checked.

That's it plain and simple. Sometimes we run around and think that something complex must be wrong when it's the miserable fact that your digestion is off, which brings us to the next section, bowels.

How often are you having a bowel movement? Do you even know how often you should be having a bowel movement? Well you should be having three to five per day if you are a woman and three a day if you are a man. What? Yep! If you don't get it out its still in, festering and putting all of those toxins back into your system. Where do you think toxins like to sit? Well they like to sit in fat cells and make them bigger and bigger and bigger and well you get the picture! A good functioning digestive tract will be a good functioning colon if you know what I mean.

Don't think that running to the store and buying laxatives will make this dream come true. As a matter of fact, laxatives can end up damaging the digestive tract and then you're stuck depending on them for life and all the while you're just full of ....

Did you know that your body actually wants to get rid of all of that stuff? Don't you feel better after a bowel movement? Come on, you know you do!

NOTES

NOTES

Glands

Moving on to the adrenal glands. Those two little glands that sit on top of the kidneys seem to manage a lot. They are responsible for helping to manage the way that glucose is used in the immune system and holding down inflammation. Then there is the balance of the minerals in the system. You know, things like magnesium, calcium, zinc, iron, things like that. Also, the innermost layer controls the sex hormones.

Tick off the adrenals and you have a fat mess. Stress in constant measure is one of the biggest ways to make those adrenal glands mad. Stress doesn't just come from the irritating person in the office next to you, it also comes from home, kids, bills and food! Yes, food.

Things you can't digest or that make your system too inflammatory can be a big time stressor. Things like alcoholic beverages, caffeine, candy, drive thru food, microwave food. All of those can tank an already stressed system and then you're down for the count, not to mention overweight. Once those adrenals have you on their hate list, you are doomed! The adrenals have three stages of fatigue.

Stage One, you recover with some rest, good food, and removing the stressor. That takes three to six months.

Stage Two is a little more intense and can take up to two years, if your body co-operates.

Then there is _Stage Three_. The poor little things are like dried up little raisins and can't function at all. There is little hope for them at this point. However, with proper nutrition and supplementation and removal of the stressors it can be done. The worst is what can happen to some people after stage three and that is Addison's Disease.

Addison's Disease is when the adrenal glands don't function at all and all of their functions must be compensated for by prescriptions, for the rest of your life. Everything will hit you extra hard and be a big project for your body. Not a good spot to be in, so take care of your adrenals!

Sometimes it's hard to tell if it's your adrenals or your thyroid that are at less than optimal functionality.

The thyroid gland is in your neck, under either your Adam's Apple or your Eve's Apple. If it's not happy it can even start to get larger and make you feel like your throat is full. Other than where it is and the fact that you've heard you can lose weight if it's running right, well, that may be all you know about it.

What you do know about yourself is that you're tired, gaining weight, and something is wrong. I think most people don't realize you can have under active thyroid symptoms before you actually have a direct diagnosis of hypothyroidism. We are all aware in this day and age that the thyroid can be responsible for feeling sluggish and getting those extra pounds to pack on around the middle, or for that matter, around the whole body.

If you are feeling tired, depressed, gaining weight, have the dry brittle nails, are constipated, maybe even feeling dizzy, you need to get your doctor involved.
One of the things that can contribute to a sluggish thyroid is your genes. A lot of times it can run in families, stay on top of your thyroid health if it runs in yours.

Other times it's a matter of stress or bad eating, which came first it's hard to say, but either way you need to get on a good eating plan because you aren't going to slim down on crunchy little candies and cookies.

The other thing about the thyroid is that it controls how you burn up the food you eat. If your thyroid is running slowly then your food gets digested slowly, if at all. If the thyroid is running too fast it can keep you up all night, doing way to many chores! (Sounds tempting but trust me, it's not good!). Either way, you can't properly use your food if the body isn't getting the right nutrition or at the right temperature to for it to burn.

Get your thyroid checked and get it checked with a complete panel.

NOTES

NOTES

CHAPTER 6

DIET IS A FOUR LETTER WORD

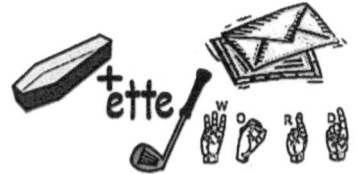

Oh, if I only had a dime for every time I was asked about the latest type of diet! How about the one where you only do 500 calories, or the one where you eat only protein, I'm an O blood type, does that work, I heard that this patch will help (Sure, put it over your mouth!). Oy! Maybe you should go on two diets because one just didn't give you enough food! LOL!

Here's the deal on diets, so listen and read closely. I don't care how many points you eat each day, what your blood type is, or what patch you put where, if your body is not in balance it won't matter. Yes, you will lose weight and think you have conquered the problem once and for all but you won't have done anything for very long. If you want to put the book down now I understand. I can wait a few minutes. Lalalala. Are you ready to start again? Done being mad and confrontational? OK.

Every person is different. Is that a shock to you? Many of the diets are places to start but they all need to be fine tuned for you! So many people lose weight and do one of two things. Either they keep it off but their optimal blood test numbers end up being horrible. They are unhealthy in the end, but hey they look good on the outside, temporarily The second possibility is they gain it back because the eating style wasn't something they could commit to for the rest of their life and their body is staging a revolt against them. Come on, you know you have been in both places, we all have.

If you are not in balance, you won't stay on the eating plan. Let me repeat it. If you are not in balance, you won't stay on the eating plan. Diet is such a weird word, don't you think. It has the ability to make us think that this is just a temporary thing done only to achieve a goal and then we can go right back to what we used to do. It's not true.

I think you need an eating plan. Yes, a plan. When you go to the grocery store most of you have a plan. What you will buy and what you will make of it or what you will

eat with it. Yes, I know it sounds so un-fun
but plans have some really great
gratification built into them. You can't just
run around willy nilly and think that you can
eat whatever you want, when you want,
how you want and achieve a goal.
Remember me saying that the diet industry
is big money? That's because they know you
will do it over and over again. If you deny
your body you will very soon reward your
body and down the slippery slope you go.

How many of you out there want to die early
after being a burden to your loved ones?
Yep, just like I thought, no hands went up.

Who wants to live a decent energized life
and just wake up when it's time, dead? Now
look at the hands that went up. In case you

were wondering, my hand went up on that last one too. That's why it's important to get yourself in balance and guess what? When you're in balance most of the junk you craved doesn't appeal anymore. You know how I know it? Because, most of you have said so and even tried it once you've gotten into balance.

It's okay to be overweight and be disappointed about it, but get yourself in balance so you can get to the real blubber of the matter. This brings me to my next point.

What's the best size to be? No it's not a college or high school weight. You've changed, let that go. How about being realistic about the whole thing? You didn't

just wake up one day over weight, did you?
There was a point where you felt
comfortable about your size. That's the
place you want to be, get a reality check for
yourself.

Healthy is not really skinny. Too many
people think so. Not true. The other
problem is people use BMI (Body Mass
Index), another bad idea. It's not accurate
for those who are more bone or muscle
dense.

If you are unsure where you should be ask
your healthcare professional for advice I'm
sure he or she will be able to properly guide
you to where you look good, feel good, and
your blood scores are in the optimal ranges.

NOTES

NOTES

CHAPTER 7

WHERE TO START

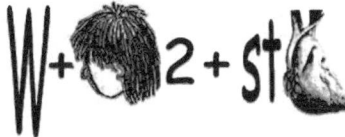

I wanted to keep this book short because too much information can make your head swim and my guess is by now your head is swimming so here is the starting point.

First of all, if your digestion is junk you can forget any diet because everything else is going to be off. If you put it in your mouth and nothing comes of it what was the point of it? Oh you may lose weight for a while but only until another deficiency pops up and creates diet duck soup, so get the digestion rolling in the right direction.

Secondly, make sure your adrenal glands aren't in the dumper. If they are in the dumper you won't be going anywhere but to the couch and the coffee shop. Neither are good for burning calories.

Third, make sure that your blood work is reflecting optimal ranges and not just functional ranges. In functional ranges you might be able to get up and breathe but you surely won't be doing it with a smile on your face! Moving toward optimal ranges will involve talking a lot about vitamin and mineral deficiencies, and we all read about those. Fourth, get either the hormones tested or the neurotransmitters tested. My money would be on the neurotransmitters since a lot of what they do is control the hormones.

Once all of those have been evaluated and it's been decided whether or not you need a stool test for digestion, ask your Naturopath to help you get a good eating plan that you can live with and then do it! Yes, I said do it. Food and weight shouldn't take over your life, you should take it over!

Next, throw out the fat clothes. You are not ten years old and going to grow into them! Get rid of them, now! Don't even hang onto a shirt or pair of pants for those days you feel heavier, donate them today.

Lastly get moving! Do something that resembles exercise and the kind of exercise I'm talking about is not just lifting the fork to your mouth. Go outside! Do something, make a difference. Break into someone's yard and rake it for them if yours is already done. (If they call the police don't come knockin' on my door!)

Find a good Naturopath. He or she will be able to guide you properly through the process.

NOTES

NOTES

About This Book

It is here at Olive Branch Wellness Center that we try to put ourselves out of business by educating the people who come t us.

The education of those people is exactly what I have been trying for years to accomplish so that everyone can live the be life they can, as opposed to being trapped in the doctor's office.

When I wrote Livin' La Vida Grande, I wanted everyone to understand that sometimes you just can't get to where you're going using the same route you've always taken. While sometimes those things work and work well, our bodies do change. Then it becomes difficult to navigate away from our habits and blaze a new path without some guidance from someone who does this all day, every day. After all, sometime it really isn't your fault. That's what we are here for at Olive Branch Wellness. Our passion is you and your health!

If you would like to get monthly newsletters from <u>Olive Brancl Wellness Center,</u> please go to the <u>Articles of Interest</u> section (<u>olivebwc.com</u> and sign up. You may also follow us on Faceboo Pinterest, LinkedIn, Twitter, and YouTube.

ABOUT THE AUTHOR

Raynette Ilg, ND

Who is this woman? Raynette Ilg graduated from National University of Health Sciences in Lombard Illinois with a Bachelors of Bio Medicine and a Doctorate of Naturopathic Medicine. Raynette Ilg is owner of Olive Branch Wellness Cent located in South Elgin, Illinois.

www.ingramcontent.com/pod-product-compliance
Lightning Source LLC
Chambersburg PA
CBHW020518290526
45786CB00002B/651